Vegan Cookbook

40+ High-Protein Plant-Based Diet - Vegan Meal Prep Cookbook to Build Strong Body, Fuel Workout, Maintain Health and Vitality

Ronnie Platt

Copyright 2020 by Ronnie Platt - All rights reserved

No part of this publication may be reproduced or transmitted in any form or by any means, mechanical or electronic, including photocopying and recording, or by any information storage and retrieval system, without permission, in written, from the author.

All attempts have been made to verify information provided in this publication. Neither the author nor the publisher assumes any responsibility for errors or omissions of the subject matter herein. This publication is not intended for use as a source of legal or accounting advice. The Publisher wants to stress that the information contained herein may be subject to varying state and/or local laws or regulations. All users are advised to retain competent counsel to determine what state and/or local laws or regulations may apply to the user's particular business.

The purchaser or reader of this publication assumes responsibility for the use of these materials and information. Adherence to all applicable laws and regulations, federal, state, and local, governing professional licensing, business practices, advertising, and all other aspects of doing business in the United States or any other jurisdiction is the sole responsibility of the purchaser or reader.

The author and Publisher assume no responsibility or liability whatsoever on the behalf of any purchaser or reader of these materials for injury due to use of any of the methods contained herein. Any perceived slights of specific people or organizations are unintentional.

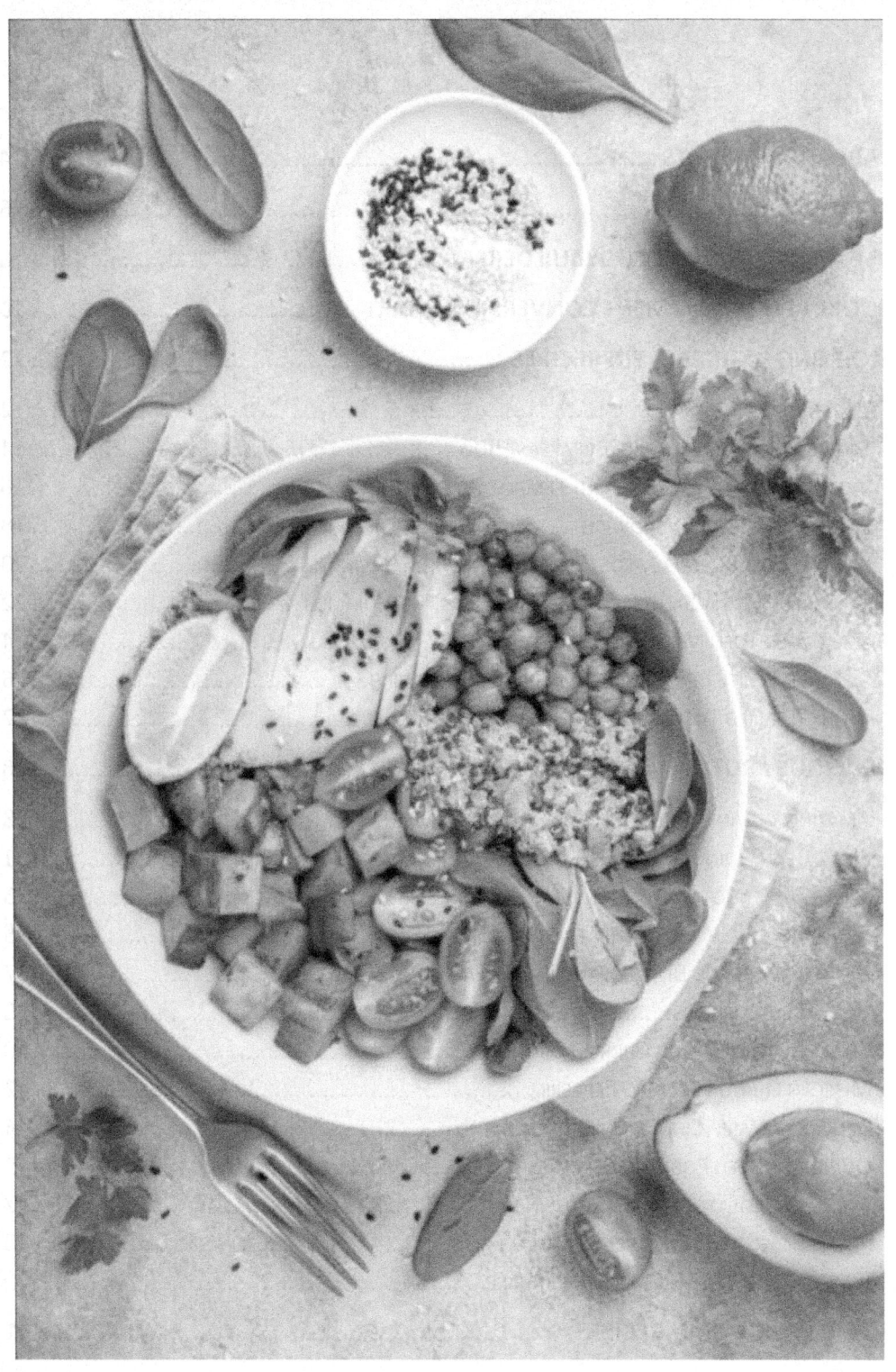

Table of Contents

TABLE OF CONTENTS 4
INTRODUCTION 6
VEGAN OPTIONS FOR BODYBUILDERS 8
COOKING MEASUREMENT CONVERSION CHART 10
MORNING HIGH-PROTEIN RECIPES 12
    VEGAN BREAKFAST SANDWICH 12
    SIMPLE CHICKPEA SCRAMBLE BREAKFAST BOWL 14
    VEGAN BUTTERNUT SQUASH AND TEMPEH TACOS 16
    DELICIOUS CHICKPEA SANDWICH 18
    SPICED SWEET POTATO TACOS 20
    FLAVORFUL VEGAN SANDWICH WITH CHICKPEAS AND HUMMUS 22
    SCRAMBLED TOFU MORNING BURRITO 24
    SMASHED WHITE BEAN, BASIL, & AVOCADO SANDWICH 26
    VEGAN CURRIED TOFU SCRAMBLE WITH SPINACH 27
DELICIOUS PROTEIN VEGAN SNACKS & SALADS 28
    AMAZING VEGAN PROTEIN BURRITO 28
    BLACK BEAN QUINOA BURGERS 31
    SPICED SWEET POTATO TACOS 33
    HIGH-PROTEIN ZUCCHINI "MEATBALLS" 35
    MOUTH-WATERING BLACK BEAN TEMPEH TACOS 37
    VEGAN LENTIL WRAPS 38
    CHICKPEA, MANGO AND CURRIED CAULIFLOWER SALAD 40
    MEXICAN QUINOA STUFFED PEPPERS 42
    DELICIOUS WARM CINNAMON QUINOA SALAD 44
    QUINOA STUFFED POBLANO PEPPERS 45
    VEGAN CHOCOLATE ALMOND PROTEIN BARS 47
    PLANT-BASED BBQ CHICKPEA SALAD 48
    JUMBO HIGH-PROTEIN CHICKPEA PANCAKE 49
PLANT-BASED MAIN RECIPES 51
    PLANT-BASED CHICKPEA NUGGETS 51

Easy Vegan Chilli Sin Carne	53
Protein Power Lentils and Amaranth Patties	55
Nourishing Veggie Bowl	56
Protein-Rich Mushroom Patties	57
Tempeh Vegetarian Chili	59
Black Bean Sweet Potato Chili	60
Savory High-Protein Coconut Lentil Curry	62
Skillet Potato and Tempeh Hash	64
The Vegan Buddha Bowl	66
Sesame Soba Noodles with Collard Greens and Tempeh Croutons	68
Vegan Chow Mein with Zucchini Noodles and Tofu	70
High-Protein Cauliflower Rice Burrito Bowl	72
Vegetarian Slow Cooker Lentil Sloppy Joes with Spaghetti Squash	74
Chickpea, Tofu, and Eggplant Curry	76
Roasted Teriyaki Mushrooms and Broccolini Soba Noodles	78
HIGH-PROTEIN SOUP & STEW RECIPES	**80**
Lentil Spinach Soup	80
Extremely Delicious Lentil Soup	82
Sweet Potato, Spinach & Butter Bean Stew	84
Pressure Cooker Pea Soup	86
CONCLUSION	**87**

Introduction

First of all, I want to say thank you for choosing my Vegan Cookbook for Athletes. In it you will find a large amount of high-protein vegan recipes that are perfect for athletes and sportsmen of all levels of training, as well as for active people who watch their health and want to dive into vegetarianism.

Today it sounds amazing, but there are many vegan bodybuilders in the world. And it sounds strange because for years big muscles in athletes have been associated with a lot of meat and eggs.

That's obvious, because muscle building comes from high protein intake. And meat, eggs and dairy products are known to be rich in protein.

But thanks to recent scientific research, as well as science in general, weightlifters and powerlifters can develop equally large muscles by sticking to plant-based foods.

This may seem like something unrealistic, but it really works. More and more athletes, not only athletes, but also fighters, boxers, runners, football players - all those who need strong muscles - are switching to plant-based meals. In addition to active muscle growth, such a diet allows to increase training productivity, increase their intensity, as well as improve performance in various sports.

If you're not a professional athlete, that's okay. A high-protein plant-based diet will make your workout more productive and also improve your health.

By the way, if you're worried that by refusing animal proteins your body will no longer get the nutrients it needs, you're wasted. Plant-based meals are very diverse and contain a lot of vitamins, minerals and trace elements that your body needs.

Vegan Options for Bodybuilders

Many people are still afraid to switch on vegetarian food as they are worried that they will lack basic nutrients: proteins, fats and carbohydrates. Below I have written a brief overview of the sources so that you have as few questions as possible.

Vegan Protein Sources

The best sources of protein are those that can be absorbed quickly and contain large amounts of amino acids. In this respect, the best source is nuts.

A mixture of almonds, pistachios and peanuts provides the body with the necessary amount of protein and calories. Also due to the fact that nuts contain a lot of useful fats and fibre, it is a great food.

Beans are another important plant source of protein, so it is a great idea to include them in your diet as well. Any bean contains a lot of protein.

Finally, there are high-protein vegetables. Spinach, kale, broccoli - all these vegetables just have to be on your table. You can make smoothies from them, use them in salads or just steam.

Vegan Fat Sources

I already mentioned nuts as a great source of fat, but there's something better: coconut oil. It's a source of unsaturated fats, which is very healthy.

Avocado is another plant fat source. This fruit contains a lot of unsaturated fats which are very useful for the cardiovascular system, brain, nervous system. Suffice it to say that avocado is a very common ingredient in vegan dishes, including for athletes.

Vegan Carbohydrate Sources

Of course, the main source of carbohydrates is porridge and cereals. Quinoa, brown rice or other grains are all great sources of slow carbohydrates.

The body also gets carbohydrates from fruits. Apple, banana, pear - all fruits are delicious and contain carbohydrates.

Finally, squashes. If it is zucchini, butternut, or a simple pumpkin, squashes are filled with nutrients and carbs.

By consuming all these ingredients in sufficient quantities, you will not be hungry, and you will receive all the necessary macro nutrients.

Cooking Measurement Conversion Chart

Liquid Measures

1 gal = 4 qt = 8 pt = 16 cups = 128 fl oz
½ gal = 2 qt = 4 pt = 8 cups = 64 fl oz
¼ gal = 1 qt = 2 pt = 4 cups = 32 fl oz
½ qt = 1 pt = 2 cups = 16 fl oz
¼ qt = ½ pt = 1 cup = 8 fl oz

Dry Measures

1 cup = 16 Tbsp = 48 tsp = 250ml
¾ cup = 12 Tbsp = 36 tsp = 175ml
⅔ cup = 10 ⅔ Tbsp = 32 tsp = 150ml
½ cup = 8 Tbsp = 24 tsp = 125ml
⅓ cup = 5 ⅓ Tbsp = 16 tsp = 75ml
¼ cup = 4 Tbsp = 12 tsp = 50ml
⅛ cup = 2 Tbsp = 6 tsp = 30ml
1 Tbsp = 3 tsp = 15ml

Dash or Pinch or Speck = less than ⅛ tsp

Quickies

1 fl oz = 30 ml
1 oz = 28.35 g
1 lb = 16 oz (454 g)
1 kg = 2.2 lb
1 quart = 2 pints

U.S.	Canadian
¼ tsp	1.25 mL
½ tsp	2.5 mL
1 tsp	5 mL
1 Tbl	15 mL
¼ cup	50 mL
⅓ cup	75 mL
½ cup	125 mL
⅔ cup	150 mL
¾ cup	175 mL
1 cup	250 mL
1 quart	1 liter

Recipe Abbreviations

Cup = c or C
Fluid = fl
Gallon = gal
Ounce = oz
Package = pkg
Pint = pt
Pound = lb or #
Quart = qt
Square = sq
Tablespoon = T or Tbl
or TBSP or TBS
Teaspoon = t or tsp

*Some measurements were rounded

Fahrenheit (°F) to Celcius (°C)
°C = (°F - 32) x 5/9

°F	°C
32°F	0°C
40°F	4°C
140°F	60°C
150°F	65°C
160°F	70°C
225°F	107°C
250°F	121°C
275°F	135°C
300°F	150°C
325°F	165°C
350°F	177°C
375°F	190°C
400°F	205°C
425°F	220°C
450°F	230°C
475°F	245°C
500°F	260°C

OVEN TEMPERATURES

WARMING: 200°F
VERY SLOW: 250°F - 275°F
SLOW: 300°F - 325°F
MODERATE: 350°F - 375°F
HOT: 400°F - 425°F
VERY HOT: 450°F - 475°F

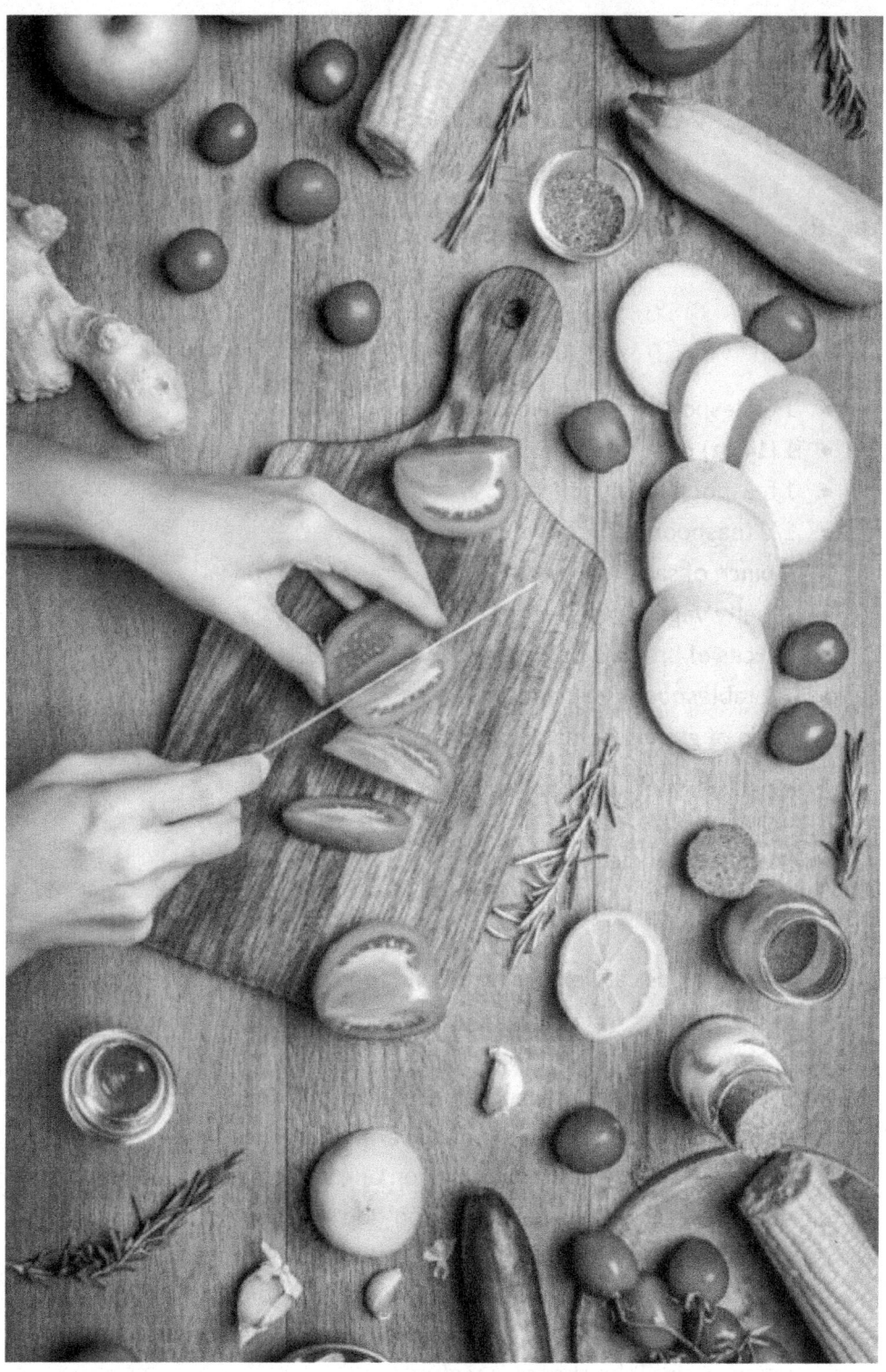

Morning High-Protein Recipes

Vegan Breakfast Sandwich

Ready in 20 minutes

Servings: 3

Ingredients

- 1 tablespoon vegetable oil
- 1 (14 oz) pack tofu, pressed & cut lengthwise into 6 even slices
- 1 teaspoon turmeric
- 1/2 teaspoon garlic powder
- A pinch of salt
- 3 melty vegan cheese slices
- 6 slices of bread, 3 or wraps
- 1-2 tablespoons vegan mayo
- 1 cup of greens (spinach, spring mix, green lettuce, etc)
- 1-2 medium tomatoes, sliced thin
- 6 pickle slices
- Fresh cracked pepper, to taste

Instructions

1. Press tofu, discard excess water and then, cut the piece lengthwise into 6 slices.
2. In a small bowl combine salt, garlic powder, turmeric and cracked pepper. Season tofu slices with this mixture from one side.
3. Heat the vegetable oil in the pan over medium heat and place tofu pieces seasoned side down. Cook on one side for about 3-5 minutes, until brown. Meanwhile, season top side with the mixture. Flip sliced and cook for another 3-5 minutes.
4. Then, melt the vegan cheese. Place 2 slices of tofu side by side, with a slice of cheese on top of each set. Put it in the oven on broil for 1-3 minutes, until the cheese is melted.

5. Spread mayo on the bread. Place the 2 slices of tofu with cheese on one side. Add the greens and tomatoes. Add a couple of pickle slices and close the sandwich together.
6. Serve and enjoy healthy vegan breakfast.

Nutrition Facts

Serving: 1sandwich | Calories: 364kcal | Carbohydrates: 51g | Protein: 16g | Fat: 12g | Saturated Fat: 5g | Sodium: 413mg | Potassium: 546mg | Fiber: 3g | Sugar: 6g | Vitamin A: 1280IU | Vitamin C: 8.4mg | Calcium: 137mg | Iron: 4.1mg

Simple Chickpea Scramble Breakfast Bowl

Ready in 20 minutes

Servings: 2 bowls

Ingredients

Chickpea Scramble

- 1 can (15 oz) chickpeas
- 1/2 Tsp turmeric
- A pinch of salt
- Freshly ground black pepper, to taste
- 1/2 small onion, diced
- 2 cloves garlic, minced
- 1-2 tbsp olive oil

Breakfast Bowl

- Mixed Greens
- Handful of parsley minced
- Handful of cilantro minced
- 1 medium-sized avocado

Instructions

Chickpea Scramble

1. In a large bowl, pour out chickpeas and a little bit of the water they're in. Mash chickpeas slightly with a fork, leaving some whole. Sprinkle with turmeric, salt, and pepper. Stir to combine well.
2. Mince garlic and dice onion. Heat the olive oil in a pan over medium-high heat. Drizzle 1 tablespoon of olive oil. Sauté the onions until they are soft. Then add minced garlic and continue sautéing until garlic is fragrant - about a minute. Mix often and don't let the garlic become brown.
3. When onions and garlic are done, add in mashed chickpeas and sauté for about five minutes.

Breakfast Bowls

1. Assemble the breakfast bowls. Add in some mixed greens at the bottom of the bowls, topped with the chickpea mixture. Top with chopped cilantro and parsley. Serve with avocado slices and enjoy.

Nutrition Facts

Calories: 355kcal | Carbohydrates: 29g | Protein: 14g | Fat: 5g | Saturated Fat: 1g | Cholesterol: 18mg

Vegan Butternut Squash and Tempeh Tacos

Ready in 15 minutes

Servings: nearly 10 tacos

Ingredients

For the tacos

- 1 pound of butternut squash, peeled and cut in 1/2-inch cubes
- 4 tbsp vegetable oil, divided
- 1 tsp cumin
- 1/2 tsp cinnamon
- A pinch of salt
- 1/4 tsp freshly ground black pepper
- 1/2 small yellow onion, chopped
- 2 large cloves garlic, minced
- 1 1/2 tbsp taco seasoning
- Juice of 1/2 lime
- 8oz package of tempeh, crumbled with hands
- 4 tbsp fresh cilantro, finely chopped
- 10 corn tortillas
- Avocado slices and lime wedges to serve

For the Salsa Verde

- 1 cup tomatillos, husks removed and rinsed
- 1 jalapeño pepper, cut in half lengthwise, veins removed
- 1 small onion, chopped
- 1 clove garlic
- 1/3 cup water
- 1/2 tsp lime juice
- A pinch of salt
- Chopped cilantro

Instructions

For the tacos

1. In a large bowl mix cubed butternut squash with 2 tbsp oil, season with cumin, cinnamon, salt and pepper. Stir to combine well. Heat large pan over medium heat and cook squash until tender, for about 10 minutes.
2. In a large saucepan, heat the oil on medium heat. Add chopped onion and cook for about 3 minutes, stirring often. Then, add garlic and cook for another couple minutes, until browned. Then, add chopped tempeh, taco seasoning, sprinkle with lime juice and cook for another 3 minutes. Add freshly chopped cilantro, stir to combine and remove from heat.
3. Cook corn tortillas over open flame on your stovetop. Cook until tortilla begins to brown, cook less then a minute. Flip and cook on other side for minute or less.
4. Assemble tacos, adding butternut squash, temper mixture and salsa. Top with avocado slices

How to cook Salsa

1. Add vegetable oil on skillet and heat over medium-high heat. Add tomatillos, chopped onion, minced garlic and jalapeno. Mix well and cook until tender for about 10 minutes.
2. When cooked, transfer all the veggies to a food processor. Add some water and pulse until smooth. Season with salt, mix well and add to tacos.
3. Enjoy.

Nutrition Facts

Calories: 412kcal | Carbohydrates: 36g | Protein: 14g | Fat: 15g | Fiber: 10g | Sugar: 5g

Delicious Chickpea Sandwich

Ready in 30 minutes

Servings: 2 sandwiches

Ingredients

Sandwich

- 1 can (15 oz) chickpeas (rinsed and drained)
- 3 tbsp sunflower seeds, roasted and unsalted
- 3 tbsp vegan mayo
- 1/2 tsp dijon or spicy mustard
- 3 tsp maple syrup
- 1 medium red onion, chopped
- 2 tbsp fresh dill, finely chopped
- 1/2 tsp salt
- A pinch of freshly ground black pepper
- 4 pieces rustic bread
- Sliced avocado, onion, tomato, for serving

Garlic Herb Sauce

- 4 tbsp hummus
- Juice of 1/2 lemon
- 1/2 tsp dried dill
- 2 large garlic cloves, minced
- Cup of water

Instructions

1. Firstly you need to prepare garlic sauce. Take a large mixing bowl and combine all sauce ingredients. Mix well, then set aside.
2. Take another large bowl, add drained chickpeas and mash with fork. Stir in sunflower seeds, mayo, mustard, maple syrup, chopped onion, dill, season with salt and pepper and stir to combine well.
3. Toast bread and prepare sandwich toppings you preference (avocado, tomato, etc)

4. Scoop a healthy amount of filling onto two of the pieces of bread, add desired toppings and sauce, and top with other two slices of bread.

Nutrition Facts

Serving: 1 sandwich without bread | Calories: 532kcal | Carbohydrates: 52g | Protein: 17g | Fat: 30g | Fiber: 14g | Sugar: 5g

Spiced Sweet Potato Tacos

Ready in 40 minutes

Servings: up to 15 tacos

Ingredients

- 1 lb sweet potato
- 1/2 medium onion, diced
- 3 garlic cloves, minced
- 1 can (15 oz) black beans, rinsed
- 1 cup frozen corn
- 1/2 tsp ground cumin
- A pinch of salt
- 1/4 tsp freshly ground black pepper
- 10-15 corn tortillas
- 1 large avocado, peeled
- 2 plum tomatoes, diced
- 2 scallions, sliced
- 4 tbsp fresh cilantro, finely chopped
- 2 tbsp freshly squeezed lemon or lime juice
- Some water

Instructions

1. Cut sweet potatoes into 1/2 inch sticks.
2. Adjust a steamer basket in a saute pan, pour in some water and bring to a simmer. Steam sweet potato sticks up to 10 minutes, until tender but not overcooked. Remove from the steamer cooker and set aside.
3. In a large skillet, add diced onion and pour in some water. Cover the lid and cook for about 5-7 minutes. Add sweet potatoes, beans, corn, season with cumin, salt and pepper. Stir to combine gently and cook over medium heat for 5-7 minutes.
4. Warm tortillas one by one for about 30 seconds in a dry skillet over high heat.
5. In a large bowl mash the avocado. Spread some avocado over the tortilla then, spoon some beans and sweet potato mixture on the top,

cover with tomatoes, scallions and cilantro. Sprinkle with some lemon juice, fold and serve.

Nutrition Facts

Serving: 1 taco | Calories 97 | Carbohydrates 10g | Fiber 4g | Protein 6g

Flavorful Vegan Sandwich with Chickpeas and Hummus

Ready in 25 minutes

Servings: 2

Ingredients

- 3 cloves garlic, minced
- 1/2 tablespoon ground cumin
- 1/2 tablespoon ground coriander
- A pinch of salt
- 1 teaspoon turmeric powder
- 1 teaspoon ground allspice
- 1/2 teaspoon ground ginger
- Freshly ground black pepper, to taste
- Pinch of cayenne pepper
- 3 tablespoons olive oil
- 1 can (15 oz), drained and rinsed
- 1/3 cup thinly sliced red onion
- 1/4 cup thinly sliced red pepper

Pita

- 2 whole wheat pita with pockets
- 1/4 cup hummus
- 1 to 2 handfuls chopped lettuce
- Fresh parsley, finely chopped, for topping

Instructions

1. In a large bowl combine garlic, cumin and pepper. Sprinkle with the olive oil, and stir to combine well. Add chickpeas, onion, red pepper. Mix evenly.
2. Preheat the oven to 400 F. Transfer chickpeas mixture to the roast pan and cover with foil. Bake on oven for about 30 minutes, until cooked.

3. Heat each pita then, spread 1 tbsp hummus on each of them. Top with lettuce and chickpea mixture. Sprinkle with freshly chopped parsley, fold and serve.

Nutrition Facts

Calories: 320kcal | Carbohydrates: 41g | Protein: 18g | Fat: 15g | Fiber: 10g | Sugar: 5g

Scrambled Tofu Morning Burrito

Ready in 30 minutes

Servings: 4

Ingredients

Tofu

- 1 package (12 oz) extra-firm tofu
- 1 tbsp vegetable oil
- 3 cloves garlic, minced
- 1 tbsp hummus
- 1/2 tsp chili powder
- 1/2 tsp cumin
- 1 tsp nutritional yeast
- A pinch of salt
- 1/4 cup minced parsley

Vegetables

- 4 whole baby potatoes (chopped into bite-size pieces)
- 1 medium red bell pepper, sliced
- 1 tbsp vegetable oil
- 1 pinch of salt
- 1/2 tsp ground cumin
- 1/2 tsp chili powder
- 2 cups chopped kale

The rest

- 3-4 large flour or gluten-free tortillas
- 1 medium ripe avocado, mashed
- Cilantro
- Chunky red or green salsa or hot sauce

Instructions

1. Preheat oven to 400 degrees F and line a baking sheet with parchment paper. Meanwhile, wrap tofu in a clean towel and set something

heavy on top to press out excess moisture. Then crumble with a fork into fine pieces. Set aside.

2. Add potatoes and red pepper to the baking sheet, drizzle with oil and spices, and toss to combine. Bake for 15-22 minutes or until fork tender and slightly browned. Add kale in the last 5 minutes of baking to wilt, tossing with the other vegetables to combine seasonings.
3. While veggies are cooking, heat a large skillet over medium heat. Sprinkle with oil, add garlic, tofu, and cook for about 10 minutes, stirring often, until brown.
4. In a medium mixing bowl, combine hummus, chili powder, cumin, nutritional yeast, season with salt, and stir to combine. Then add water until a pourable sauce is formed. Then add parsley and stir well. Add the spice mixture to the tofu and continue cooking over medium heat until slightly browned - 3-5 minutes. Set aside.
5. Assemble burritos: Roll out a large tortilla. Add generous portions of the roasted vegetables, scrambled tofu, avocado, cilantro, and a bit of salsa. Roll up and place seam side down. Continue until all toppings are used up - about 3-4 large burritos.

Nutrition Facts

Serving: buritto | Calories: 441kcal | Carbohydrates: 54g | Protein: 17g | Fat: 19g | Saturated Fat: 5g | Sodium: 772mg | Fiber: 8g | Sugar: 3,5g

Smashed White Bean, Basil, & Avocado Sandwich

Ready in 5-7 minutes

Servings: 4

Ingredients

- 8 whole-grain bread slices
- 1 heaped tablespoon whole grain dijon mustard
- Salt and pepper to taste
- 1 15 oz can white beans, drained and rinsed
- 1 avocado, sliced
- Juice of half a lemon
- 2 tablespoons fresh basil leaves, finely chopped
- For the sandwich (optional): baby spinach, romaine, arugula, tomato slices

Instructions

1. Pour white beans into a large bowl and mashed a little with a potato masher. Add in the diced avocado and lemon juice, then mash until there are just a few chunks of bean and avocado left. Stir in the mustard, basil, salt and pepper, then taste and adjust flavors as necessary.
2. Spoon onto a sandwich, salad, veggie bowl, or just eat it as is! It's delicious any way!

Nutrition Facts

Serving: 1 sandwich | Calories: 285kcal | Carbohydrates: 28g | Protein: 12g | Fat: 8g | Fiber: 3g | Sugar: 2g

Vegan Curried Tofu Scramble with Spinach

Ready in 20 minutes

Servings: 2

Ingredients

- 1 teaspoon olive oil
- 1 medium-sized onion, diced
- 3 cloves garlic, minced
- 1 container firm tofu, pressed and crumbled
- 1 teaspoon curry powder
- 1/2 teaspoon turmeric
- Salt and pepper, to taste
- 2 tomatoes, diced
- 1 bunch fresh spinach

Instructions

1. Heat the skillet over medium-high heat. Sprinkle with the olive oil and sauté garlic with onion for about 4-5 minutes. Stir in crumbled tofu and stir well. Season with curry powder, turmeric, salt and pepper. Mix well.
2. The next step, add diced tomatoes and cook more, stirring often.
3. Add the spinach, cover the pan and cook for 1 to 2 minutes, just until the spinach is wilted, stirring well.

Nutrition Facts

Calories: 438kcal | Carbohydrates: 48g | Protein: 34g | Fat: 17g | Fiber: 10g | Sugar: 5g

Delicious Protein Vegan Snacks & Salads

Amazing Vegan Protein Burrito

Ready in 40 minutes

Servings: 4

Ingredients

For the Quinoa

- 3/4 cup white quinoa, thoroughly rinsed
- Couple cups water
- 1/4 teaspoon sea salt
- 1 can (15 oz) black beans, drained and rinsed
- 4 tbsp chopped fresh cilantro
- 3 tablespoons lime juice, freshly squeezed
- 3 tablespoons hemp seeds
- A pinch of salt
- Freshly ground black pepper, to taste

For Kale

- 3 cups kale, destemmed and chopped
- 1 tablespoon lime juice
- 1 tbsp olive oil
- Sea salt, to taste
- Freshly ground black pepper, to taste

For the Pico de Gallo

- 1 cup quartered cherry tomatoes
- 1/4 cup finely diced red onion
- 2 tablespoons chopped cilantro
- Sea salt, to taste

For the Guacamole

- 1 ripe avocado, halved, pitted, and peeled
- 1 lime, juiced
- Sea salt, to taste

Additional Ingredients

- 4 large sprouted-grain or gluten-free tortillas

Instructions

For the Quinoa

1. In a small pot pour in water and add quinoa. Season with sea salt. Heat over medium-high heat until boiling. Reduce heat, cover, and simmer for 10-14 minutes or until quinoa is tender and translucent. Fluff with a fork and transfer to a large bowl.
2. Add the black beans, chopped cilantro, lime juice, hemp seeds, sea salt, and black pepper to the quinoa and stir. Set aside.

For the Kale

1. In a large mixing bowl, add chopped kale, sprinkle with lime juice, olive oil, and sea salt to a large mixing bowl and mix well for 2-3 minutes or until tender. Set aside.

For the Pico de Gallo

1. In a medium sized bowl mix cherry tomatoes, red onion, cilantro, and sea salt. Stir to combine and set aside.

For the Guacamole

1. Scoop the flesh of the avocado into a small bowl along with the juice of one lime and sea salt, to taste. Use the back of a fork to smash the avocado to desired consistency. Set aside.

To Assemble the Burritos

1. Lay one tortilla flat on a clean work surface. Fill the tortilla with the quinoa mixture, pico de gallo, guacamole, and kale. Begin rolling the burrito away from you, being sure to tuck the sides in as you go. Slice in half and serve immediately. Repeat.

Nutrition Facts

Serving: Calories: 522kcal | Carbohydrates: 77g | Protein: 22g | Fat: 17g | Sodium: 405mg | Sugar: 7g

Black Bean Quinoa Burgers

Ready in 1 hour

Servings: 10 burger patties

Ingredients

- 2 tablespoons flax meal + 5 tablespoons water
- 1-2 tbsp Olive oil
- 1/2 cup uncooked quinoa
- 1 small yellow onion, finely chopped
- 1 orange bell pepper, finely chopped
- 1 jalapeno pepper, seeds removed, finely chopped
- 1 tablespoon garlic, minced
- 1 cup packed spinach, chopped
- 1 1/2 cups cooked black beans, drained, or 1 can black beans, rinsed and drained
- Salt to taste
- 1 teaspoon paprika
- 1/2 teaspoon cumin
- 1/2 teaspoon pepper
- 1/8 teaspoon ground cayenne
- 1/2 cup oat flour

Instructions

1. In a medium bowl combine flax meal and water. Mix well and set aside.
2. To cook quinoa, heat 1 teaspoon of oil in a small saucepan over medium heat. Rinse quinoa in a small mesh strainer. Once oil is hot, add quinoa to the saucepan and stir. Cook for 1-2 minutes until lightly toasted. Add 1 cup water; turn the heat to high. Once boiling, reduce heat to low, cover, and simmer for 13-15 minutes.
3. Meanwhile, heat 1 tablespoon of oil in a skillet over medium heat. Once hot, add chopped onion and cook for a few minutes, stirring often. Add bell pepper, jalapeño, and garlic; cook until the onion is

translucent, about 2 minutes. Add the spinach and stir immediately, letting it wilt slightly. Turn the heat off.
4. In a large bowl mix black beans. Mash with a fork, leaving some texture. Add cooked quinoa, sautéed vegetables, salt, paprika, cumin, pepper, cayenne, and reserved flax eggs. Mix until combined, then add oat flour. Stir to combine well.
5. Preheat oven to 375F. Form 10-12 patties depending on desired size. Place on baking sheet and cook for 20 minutes, flip once and then bake for 25-30 more minutes, until browned and crispy.
6. Serve on a whole-wheat hamburger bun with guacamole, barbecue sauce, and other desired toppings, or on top of a salad.

Nutrition Facts

Serving: 1 burger patty | Calories: 114kcal | Carbohydrates: 21g | Protein: 12g | Fat: 6g | Fiber: 10g | Sugar: 2g

Spiced Sweet Potato Tacos

Ready in 40 minutes

Servings: up to 15 tacos

Ingredients

- 1 pound sweet potato
- ½ small red onion, cut into ¼-inch dice (about 1/2 cup)
- 2 small garlic cloves, minced
- 1 (15-ounce) can pinto or black beans, rinsed and drained
- ½ cup frozen sweet corn kernels, rinsed
- ½ teaspoon ground cumin
- ½ teaspoon ground ancho chile, or to taste
- Sea salt, to taste
- Up to 15 corn tortillas
- 1 ripe Hass avocado, pitted and peeled
- 2 Roma (plum) tomatoes, cored and cut into ¼-inch dice (about 1 cup)
- 3 scallions, white and green parts, thinly sliced (about 3/4 cup)
- ¼ cup finely chopped fresh cilantro
- 2 tablespoons fresh lime juice (from 1 lime)

Instructions

1. Cut the sweet potato lengthwise into 1/2 to 3/4-inch thick sticks.
2. Place a steamer basket in a sauté pan, and add 1 to 2 inches of water to the pan. Cover and bring to a simmer. Place the sweet potato wedges in the steamer, cover, and steam until the sweet potato is cooked through but not too soft, 7 to 10 minutes, making sure not to overcook. Remove the sweet potato from the pot and set aside.
3. In a large skillet, place the onion, garlic, and 2 tablespoons water. Cover and cook over low heat until the onion is translucent, about 10 minutes.
4. Add the reserved sweet potato, beans, corn, cumin, ancho chile, and salt to taste. Gently fold to coat the sweet potato with the spices. Cook over medium-low heat until heated through, 5 to 7 minutes. Remove from the heat.

5. Line a plate with a damp large, clean dish towel. Warm the tortillas one at a time for about 20 seconds on each side in a dry skillet set over medium heat. Or, if you have a gas stove, place a tortilla straight over the flame for a few seconds on each side. As you heat the tortillas, stack them on the damp towel and cover the tops of them with the towel to retain moisture.
6. Place the avocado in a small bowl and use a fork to gently mash it.
7. To form the taco, spread some avocado on half of each tortilla. Spoon some beans and sweet potato on top, and then add the tomato, scallions, and cilantro. Drizzle with some lime juice. Fold each tortilla in half. Serve at once.

Nutrition Facts

Serving: 1 taco | Calories 97 | Carbohydrates 10g | Fiber 4g | Protein 6g

High-Protein Zucchini "Meatballs"

Ready in 45 minutes

Servings: 10-12 balls

Ingredients

- 1 (15-ounce) can chickpeas, drained and rinsed
- 3 garlic cloves
- 1/2 cup rolled oats
- 1 teaspoon dried basil
- 1 teaspoon dried oregano
- 1/2 teaspoon salt
- 2 tablespoons nutritional yeast
- juice of 1/2 lemon
- 1 cup shredded zucchini (about 1 large zucchini)
- 32 ounces marinara
- 8 ounces whole grain pasta

Instructions

1. In the bowl of a food processor, combine the drained and rinsed chickpeas, garlic cloves, and rolled oats. Pulse for about 5-10 seconds, until finely chopped. When you press the mixture between your fingers, it should hold together. Transfer to a large bowl along with the dried herbs, salt, nutritional yeast, lemon juice and shredded zucchini. Do not use more than 1 cup of shredded zucchini. Stir together until well-combined. If the mixture is too wet to handle, add a little flour (you can grind extra oats into a flour) or nutritional yeast to help absorb excess moisture.
2. Preheat the oven to 375°F then line a baking sheet with parchment paper. Using your hands, scoop out on heaping tablespoon of the zucchini mixture at a time and roll into 12 separate balls. Arrange on the baking sheet a few inches apart then bake in the oven for 25 minutes. Meanwhile, cook pasta as directed.

3. Once the zucchini balls are light golden brown, remove them from the oven and set aside. Serve warm over cooked pasta with marinara sauce. Garnish with fresh basil and enjoy!

Nutrition Facts

Serving: 1 "meatball" | Calories: 53kcal | Carbohydrates: 12g | Protein: 6g | Fat: 1g | Fiber: 7g | Sugar: 2g

Mouth-Watering Black Bean Tempeh Tacos

Ready in 30 minutes

Servings: 8-10 tecos

Ingredients

- 8 oz. tempeh
- 15 oz. can black beans
- 1/2 onion, diced
- 2 cloves garlic, minced
- 2 Tbsp. taco seasoning
- Corn tortillas
- Toppings of choice: nutritional yeast, pico de gallo, lettuce, tomato, cilantro, avocado/guacamole, etc.

Instructions

1. Crumble tempeh and place in a bowl. Mix the taco seasoning with 2-3 tbsp. water and add to tempeh. Stir well to combine and set aside to marinate.
2. In a pan over medium heat, saute onion and tempeh for about 8-10 minutes. After onions have softened, add minced garlic to the pan and cook 30 seconds.
3. Add black beans (rinsed and drained) and cook about 3 minutes or until heated through.
4. Assemble tacos: warm the corn tortillas if desired, add the tempeh mixture, and any toppings.

Nutrition Facts

Calories: 151kcal | Carbohydrates: 19g | Protein: 11g | Fat: 4g | Potassium: 387mg | Fiber: 5g | Sugar: 1g

Vegan Lentil Wraps

Ready in 20 minutes

Servings: 6-8 tacos

Ingredients

Lentil filling

- 2 cups of lentils – soak over night (
- 2 small onions
- 2 garlic cloves
- 2 tbsp olive oil
- 2 tbsp dried hot paprika
- Handful basil leaves
- Handful of cilantro (or other herbs)
- Sesame seeds
- Salt to taste

For the wraps add

- Tortilla
- Broccoli roasted for 1 minute
- Roasted peppers
- Avocado dill dip

Instructions

1. Rinse soaked lentils and cook in a large deep non-stick pan at medium high heat with some water (lentils should just be covered). Make sure you stir from time to time and after about 10 minutes the lentils should be cooked. Remove water, if there is still water in the pan.
2. Meanwhile, do some preparations – chop onions, garlic, basil and cilantro.
3. After the lentils are tender and you've removed the water from the pan, add the olive oil, a pinch or two of salt, hot paprika, onions and garlic, stir in well and cook for 2-3 minutes. Turn off heat, add the rest of the ingredients – sesame seeds, cilantro, basil. Stir in everything well. Taste and add salt if you need to.

4. And now let's get to wrapping.
5. Take a big tortilla and fill it generously with the lentil filling.
6. Put some fresh and roasted vegetables on top of the lentil filling, some garlic sauce, for example my avocado dip or this spicy vegan cream cheese – wrap it and eat, even if you make a mess all over your plate and your clothing (you can also just use this bib while eating and be on the safe site).

Nutrition Facts

Calories: 418kcal | Carbohydrates: 36g | Protein: 22g | Fat: 15g | Fiber: 10g | Sugar: 5g

Chickpea, Mango and Curried Cauliflower Salad

Ready in 35 minutes

Servings: 2

Ingredients

- 1 teaspoon curry powder
- 1 teaspoon sugar
- 1 teaspoon ground mustard
- 1/2 teaspoon ground turmeric
- 1/2 teaspoon ground cumin
- 3 tablespoons olive oil
- 1 large onion, sliced
- 1 cup (15 oz) chickpeas, drained and rinsed
- 3 cups of cauliflower, cut into 1-inch florets
- 2 large mangoes peeled, pitted and chopped into 1/2-inch pieces
- 1 jalapeno stemmed, seeded and diced small
- 1 cup chopped cilantro
- 2 tablespoons lime juice
- 2 cups baby spinach
- 1 cup baby arugula
- Salt and black pepper

Instructions

1. In a small bowl, mix the curry powder, sugar, ground mustard, coriander, turmeric, cumin, salt and black pepper. Stir to combine and set aside.
2. In a large nonstick skillet, add the olive oil. Add the onion and cook for about 6 minutes over high heat. Add the spice mix and turn the heat down to medium-low. Cook for another 6 minutes. Transfer to a large bowl, and add the chickpeas to the same bowl. Leave the pan over medium heat.
3. Add the cauliflower to the same pan that cooked the onion. Add more olive oil if needed. Cook for about 5 minutes or until the cauliflower is

coated in the remaining spice mixture and is cooked through. Transfer the cauliflower to the bowl with the onion and chickpeas. Let sit at room temperature for about 20 minutes.

4. Stir in the mango, jalapeno, cilantro, lime juice, spinach and arugula. Toss so that the ingredients are evenly dispersed. Adjust seasoning to taste and serve immediately.

Nutrition Facts

Calories: 438kcal | Carbohydrates: 38g | Protein: 18g | Fat: 15g | Fiber: 8g | Sugar: 6g

Mexican Quinoa Stuffed Peppers

Ready in 1 hour

Servings: 2-3

Ingredients

Peppers

- 1 cup quinoa or rice (thoroughly rinsed and drained)
- 2 small cups vegetable stock
- 4 large red, yellow, or orange bell peppers (halved, seeds removed)
- 1/2 cup salsa (plus more for serving)
- 1 Tbsp nutritional yeast (optional)
- 2 tsp cumin powder
- 1 1/2 tsp chili powder
- 1 1/2 tsp garlic powder
- 1 15-ounce can black beans, drained
- 1 cup whole kernel corn, drained
- Toppings optional
- 1 ripe avocado (sliced)
- Fresh lime juice

Hot sauce

- Cilantro (chopped)
- Diced red onion
- Creamy Cilantro Dressing
- Chipotle Red Salsa (or your favorite salsa)

Instructions

1. Add quinoa and vegetable stock to a saucepan and bring to a boil over high heat. Once boiling, reduce heat, cover, and simmer until all liquid is absorbed and quinoa is fluffy – about 20 minutes.
2. Preheat oven to 375 degrees F and lightly grease a 9×13 baking dish or rimmed baking sheet.
3. Brush halved peppers with a neutral, high heat oil, such as avocado oil or refined coconut oil.

4. Add cooked quinoa to a large mixing bowl and add remaining ingredients – salsa through corn. Mix to thoroughly combine then taste and adjust seasonings accordingly, adding salt, pepper, or more spices as desired.
5. Generously stuff halved peppers with quinoa mixture until all peppers are full, then cover the dish with foil.
6. Bake for 30 minutes covered. Then remove foil, increase heat to 400 degrees F, and bake for another 15-20 minutes, or until peppers are soft and slightly golden brown. For softer peppers, bake 5-10 minutes more.
7. Serve with desired toppings or as is.

Nutrition Facts

Per Serving (1 of 4) | Calories: 311 | Fat: 3.4g | Sodium: 498mg | Carbohydrates: 59g | Fiber: 12g | Sugar: 8g | Protein: 15g

Delicious Warm Cinnamon Quinoa Salad

Ready in 15 minutes

Servings: 2

Ingredients

- 1 cup plant-based low fat milk
- 1 cup water
- 1 cup organic quinoa, rinsed
- 2 cups fresh blackberries
- A pinch of ground cinnamon
- 1/3 cup chopped pecans, toasted
- 4 teaspoons organic agave nectar

Instructions

1. In a medium-sized saucepan, combine plant-based milk and water. Add quinoa and bring brong to a boil over high heat. Reduce heat and cook for about 15-18 minutes, until the liquid is absorbed. Turn off heat; let stand covered 5 minutes.
2. Place blackberries to a large bowl. Sprinkle with cinnamon and stir to combine. Transfer to four bowls and top with pecans. Drizzle 1 teaspoon agave nectar over each serving.
3. While the quinoa cooks, roast the pecans in a 350F degree toaster oven for 5 to 6 minutes or in a dry skillet over medium heat for about 3 minutes.

Nutrition Facts

Calories: 410kcal | Carbohydrates: 35g | Protein: 15g | Fat: 4g

Quinoa Stuffed Poblano Peppers

Ready in 50 minutes

Servings: 4

Ingredients

- 4 poblano peppers
- 2 teaspoons olive oil, divided, plus more for the peppers
- 3/4 cup red quinoa
- 1 cup low sodium vegetable broth
- 1 medium yellow onion, chopped
- 1 garlic clove, chopped
- 1/2 cup cooked corn, thawed if frozen
- 1 cup low sodium canned black beans, rinsed and drained
- 1 4 ounce can mild diced green chiles
- 1 teaspoon chili powder
- 1/2 teaspoon ground cumin
- A pinch of salt and freshly ground black pepper
- 3 tablespoons cotija cheese
- Chopped fresh cilantro, optional
- Plain 0% fat Greek yogurt, optional

Instructions

1. Preheat the broiler to high and place an oven rack in the second from the top position.
2. Rub poblanos with olive oil and place in a well seasoned cast iron skillet or oiled oven safe baking dish. Broil until the skin of the pepper is blistered and beginning to brown, 5-10 minutes per side. Remove the peppers from the oven and place them in a bowl. Cover the top tightly with plastic wrap and allow to rest for 5-10 minutes. Move the oven rack down to the middle position and heat the oven to 375ºF.
3. Meanwhile, place quinoa in a fine mesh strainer and rinse under cold water for 2 minutes. In a medium sized pot, heat 1 teaspoon olive oil over medium heat. Once hot, add the quinoa and toast, stirring, for 1 minute. Add vegetable broth and 1/2 cup water. Bring to a boil, cover,

and reduce heat to medium low. Allow the quinoa to cook undisturbed until all of the liquid is absorbed, about 15 minutes. Remove from the heat and allow the quinoa to sit, covered, another 5 minutes.
4. Heat 1 teaspoon olive oil in a small skillet over medium heat. Once hot, add the onions and garlic. Cook, stirring often, until softened and just beginning to brown, 5-7 minutes.
5. In a large bowl, combine quinoa, onions, garlic, corn, beans, green chiles, chili powder, cumin, and salt and pepper to taste.
6. Remove the peppers from the bowl and remove skins. They should peel off easily, but don't worry about getting every last bit off. Carefully cut each pepper in half and remove the seeds. Arrange peppers cut side up in the same dish you broiled them in. Fill them evenly with the quinoa mixture and sprinkle with the cotija cheese.
7. Bake the stuffed peppers in the oven until heated through, about 15 minutes. Sprinkle with chopped cilantro and drizzle with yogurt if desired and serve.

Nutrition Facts

Calories: 292kcal | Carbohydrates: 46g | Protein: 12g | Fat: 7g | Saturated Fat: 2g | Cholesterol: 11mg | Sodium: 533mg

Vegan Chocolate Almond Protein Bars

Ready in 20 minutes

Servings: 12 bars

Ingredients

- 6 oz raw almonds
- 1/4 teaspoon sea salt
- 1 teaspoon cinnamon
- 6 oz rolled oats
- 6 oz plant-based vanilla protein powder
- 4 fl oz maple syrup
- 2 oz dairy-free chocolate chips

Instructions

1. Prepare an eight-by-eight-inch square pan by lining it with parchment paper or cooking spray.
2. Measure out 2 oz of the almonds, chop, and set aside for the topping.
3. In a food processor, pour in the remaining almonds and salt. Process until you have almond butter, or several minutes.
4. Add the oats, protein powder, cinnamon, and maple syrup, and process until smooth.
5. Press the mixture into the pan using the back of a spoon. Top with the chopped almonds, pressing those into the bars.
6. Place the chocolate chips in a small glass bowl, and microwave until melted. Drizzle the chocolate over the bars, and allow to set in the fridge for 20 minutes before cutting.
7. Store the uneaten bars in an airtight container in the fridge.

Nutrition Facts

Serving: 1 bar | Calories: 166kcal | Carbohydrates: 18g | Protein: 13g | Fat: 6g | Saturated Fat: 1.2g | Sodium: 162mg | Fiber: 3g | Sugar: 7g

Plant-Based BBQ Chickpea Salad

Ready in 18 minutes

Servings: 4

Ingredients

- 1 19 oz can chickpeas (2 cups), drained and rinsed
- 1/2 cup of your favourite vegan BBQ Sauce
- 6 cups romaine lettuce (two romaine hearts), chopped
- 1 cup cherry tomatoes, halved
- 1 cup cucumber, sliced
- 1 cup corn kernel (fresh or frozen and thawed)
- 1/4 red onion, thinly sliced
- 6 Tablespoons Vegan Creamy Ranch Dressing
- Lime wedges for garnish

Instructions

1. Add the chickpeas to a saucepan with the BBQ sauce and put over medium heat. Let the chickpeas simmer in the sauce for about 5 to 10 minutes until the sauce thickens and sticks to the chickpeas. Remove from heat and set aside.
2. Divide the lettuce among two large bowls. Then divide all of the vegetable and the BBQ chickpeas on top of the lettuce. I like to pile each ingredient in its own section so it looks pretty, but you can arrange it however you like. Drizzle with creamy vegan ranch dressing and garnish with a wedge of lime.

Nutrition Facts

Calories: 457kcal | Carbohydrates: 57g | Protein: 11g | Fat: 12g | Saturated Fat: 3g | Sodium: 549mg | Potassium: 928mg | Fiber: 6g | Sugar: 6g

Jumbo High-Protein Chickpea Pancake

Ready in 20 minutes

Servings: 1 large pancake

Ingredients

- 1 green onion, finely chopped (about 1/4 cup)
- 1/4 cup finely chopped red pepper
- 1/2 cup chickpea flour
- 1/4 teaspoon garlic powder
- 1/4 teaspoon fine grain sea salt
- 1/8 teaspoon freshly ground black pepper
- 1/4 teaspoon baking powder
- 1/2 cup + 2 tablespoons water
- For serving: salsa, avocado, hummus, cashew cream (optional)

Instructions

1. Prepare the vegetables and set aside. Preheat a 10-inch skillet over medium heat.
2. In a small bowl, whisk together the chickpea flour, garlic powder, salt, pepper, baking powder.
3. Add the water and whisk well until no clumps remain. I like to whisk it for a good 15 seconds to create lots of air bubbles in the batter. Stir in the chopped vegetables.
4. When the skillet is pre-heated (a drop of water should sizzle on the pan), spray it liberally with olive oil or other non stick cooking spray.
5. Pour on all of the batter (if making 1 large pancake) and quickly spread it out all over the pan. Cook for about 5-6 minutes on one side (timing will depend on how hot your pan is), until you can easily slide a pancake flipper/spatula under the pancake and it's firm enough not to break when flipping. Flip pancake carefully and cook for another 5 minutes, until lightly golden. Be sure to cook for enough time as this pancake takes much longer to cook compared to regular pancakes.
6. Serve on a large plate and top with your desired toppings. Leftovers can be wrapped up and placed in the fridge. Reheat on a skillet until warmed throughout.

Nutrition Facts

1 Serving Calories: 100kcal | Carbohydrates: 15g | Protein: 7g | Fat: 1.5g | Saturated Fat 0g| Fiber: 3g | Sugar: 4g

Plant-Based Main Recipes

Plant-based Chickpea Nuggets

Ready in 30 minutes

Servings: 4

Ingredients

- 1/2 cup panko breadcrumbs
- 1/2 cup rolled oats
- 1 can (15 oz) garbanzo beans (do not drain)
- A pinch of salt to taste
- 1/2 teaspoon garlic powder
- 1/2 teaspoon onion powder

Instructions

1. Arrange a rack in the middle of the oven and heat to 375°F.
2. Place the panko on a rimmed baking sheet and bake until toasted and golden-brown, about 5 minutes. Transfer to a large bowl and set aside to cool while preparing the nuggets. Line the baking sheet with parchment paper.
3. Place the oats in a food processor fitted with the blade attachment and process into a fine flour. Transfer to a large bowl and reserve the food processor.
4. Drain the chickpeas over a bowl or measuring cup, then, save the chickpeas and 1/4 cup of the liquid. Place the chickpeas into the food processor; Season with salt, garlic, and onion powder; and pulse until crumbly. Keep mixture in the food processor.
5. In a large mixing bowl whisk 1/4 cup of the chickpea liquid until foamy. Add the foamy chickpea liquid and 1/2 cup of the oat flour to the food processor. Pulse until the mixture forms a ball. You may have a little oat flour leftover, which you can add to the chickpea mixture 1 tablespoon at a time if the mixture is loose.
6. Divide the chickpea mixture into 12 equal portions and shape each one into a nugget. Coat each nugget completely in the toasted panko and place on the parchment-lined baking sheet.

7. Bake until crispy, 15 to 20 minutes. Serve warm with your favorite dipping sauce.

Nutrition Facts

Serving: Calories: 205kcal | Carbohydrates: 35g | Protein: 10g | Fat: 4g | Sodium: 289mg | Sugar: 4g

Easy Vegan Chilli Sin Carne

Ready in 40 minutes

Servings: 6

Ingredients

- 2 tbsp olive oil
- 3 cloves of garlic, minced
- 1 large red onion, thinly sliced
- 2 celery stalks, finely chopped
- 2 medium carrots, peeled and finely chopped
- 2 red peppers, roughly chopped
- 1 tsp ground cumin
- 1 tsp chili powder
- Salt and pepper, to taste
- 1 1/2 pound tinned chopped tomatoes
- 1 pound tin of red kidney beans, drained and rinsed
- 4 oz split red lentils
- 1 pound frozen soy mince
- 2 cups vegetable stock

Optional add-ins

- 1 tsp miso paste
- 2 tbsp balsamic vinegar
- A large handful of fresh coriander, roughly chopped

For Serving

- Cooked basmati rice
- Extra chopped coriander
- A squeeze of lime juice

Instructions

1. Heat the olive oil in a large saucepan. Add in garlic, onion, celery, carrots and peppers, and saute for a few minutes, on a medium heat, until softened.

2. Add the cumin, chilli powder, salt and pepper and stir.
3. Pour in the chopped tomatoes, kidney beans, lentils, soy mince and vegetable stock. Simmer for 25 minutes.
4. Serve with some steamed basmati rice, some fresh torn coriander and a squeeze of lime juice. Enjoy!

Nutrition Facts

Calories 340 | Carbohydrates 42g | Fiber 18g | Protein 25g

Protein Power Lentils and Amaranth Patties

Ready in 35 minutes

Servings: nearly 15 patties

Ingredients

- 1 cup red lentils
- ½ cup amaranth
- ½ cup chopped fresh parsley
- 1 medium-sized onion, diced
- 2 tbsp psyllium husks (or one large egg)
- 4 tbsp nutritional yeast
- ½ cup panko breadcrumbs
- Couple sliced black olives (optional)
- A pinch of salt
- Freshly ground black pepper, to taste
- 2 tbsp olive oil

Instructions

1. Add red lentils and amaranth in a pot. Pour in water bring to a boil. Simmer for 15 minutes. Strain them. Then, put them in a large bowl and blend in all the other ingredients, except oil. If the composition is too moist, add more breadcrumbs. The patties should be easy to form.
2. Heat some oil in a non-stick frying pan over medium-high heat.
3. Make the patties – 1 tbsp per patty. Fry them 2 minutes on each side.
4. Put the amaranth patties on a plate covered with a paper towel, in order to absorb all excess oil.
5. Serve and enjoy.

Nutrition Facts

Servings 1 patty | Calories 97 | Carbohydrates 10g | Fiber 4g | Protein 6g

Nourishing Veggie Bowl

Ready in 10 minutes

Servings: 2

Ingredients

- 1 cup cooked brown rice (or any grain you prefer)
- 1 ripe avocado, sliced
- 1/3 cup carrots, grated or chopped
- 4 radishes, sliced
- 1/2 cup snap peas, raw or steamed
- 1/2 cup fava beans, cooked
- 1/2 cup Cleveland Kraut Beet Red

Instructions

1. Divide each ingredient between 2 serving bowls. Mix ingredients well.
2. Sprinkle veggies with lemon juice, olive oil or tahini dressing.

Nutrition Facts

Calories: 312kcal | Carbohydrates: 35g | Protein: 13g | Fat: 4g | Saturated Fat: 1g | Cholesterol: 11mg | Sodium: 533mg

Protein-Rich Mushroom Patties

Ready in 30 minutes

Servings: 15 patties

Ingredients

- 4 cups button mushrooms, chopped
- 5 Tbsp hemp seeds
- 3 Tbsp dill, chopped
- 1 onion, chopped
- 2 tsp dry thyme
- 2 Tbsp ground flax seeds+ 3 Tbsps water (or one large egg)
- 4 Tbsp nutritional yeast
- 3-4 Tbsp hemp protein powder
- 4 Tbsp white wine
- 3 Tbsp oil for frying/baking + 1 Tbsp oil for cooking
- Sea salt and ground black pepper, to taste

Instructions

1. Mix the ground flax and water in a small bowl and set aside for 5 minutes to thicken.
2. Meanwhile, heat 1 Tbsp of oil in a large skillet. Add chopped onion and saute for 2 minutes.
3. Add chopped mushrooms, dry thyme, wine, salt, and pepper. Saute for 10 minutes and cover with a lid. Remove from heat.
4. Add egg/flax egg and inactive dry yeast flakes and mix al ingredients together. Add chopped dill, hemp seeds and hemp protein powder. When adding hemp protein powder, start by adding 3 Tbsps. If the composition is too moist and you cannot make the patties easily, add more until it has the right consistency. The hemp powder will absorb all excess water.
5. Grease a non-stick pan with some oil and add the patties - 1tbsp per patty. Fry 1-2 minutes on each side.
6. Serve and enjoy.

Nutrition Facts

Serving: 1 patty | Calories: 87kcal | Carbohydrates: 12g | Protein: 13g | Fat: 4g | Saturated Fat: 1g | Sodium: 533mg

Tempeh Vegetarian Chili

Ready in 30 minutes

Servings: 4

Ingredients

- 2 Tbsp olive oil
- 1 8-oz package tempeh, roughly grated
- 1 medium white onion diced
- 1 red bell pepper diced
- 1 stalk celery diced
- 2 cloves garlic minced
- 3/4 cup tomato sauce
- 1 15-oz can kidney beans, drained
- 1 15-oz can black beans, drained
- 1 cup water
- 1 tsp each cumin and salt
- 1/4 tsp each chili powder and crushed red pepper flakes
- Chopped green onions, plain Greek yogurt, for serving

Instructions

1. Heat oil over medium/high heat in a large pot. Add tempeh and cook until lightly browned, about 5 minutes. It's okay if some of it sticks to the bottom of the pan. It will come off when you add the liquids.
2. Add onion, bell pepper, celery, and garlic, continuing to cook until veggies are a bit soft, about 5 minutes.
3. Add the remaining ingredients, reduce heat to medium, and cook until warm and the flavors have blended, about 15 minutes. Taste and adjust seasonings as needed. Top with green onions and serve.

Nutrition Facts

Serving: 1serving | Calories: 522kcal | Carbohydrates: 64g | Protein: 30g | Fat: 22g | Sodium: 1900mg | Fiber: 17g

Black Bean Sweet Potato Chili

Ready in 50 minutes

Servings: 4

Ingredients

- 1 tablespoon plus 2 teaspoons olive oil
- 1 medium-large sweet potato peeled and diced
- 1 large red onion diced
- 4 cloves garlic minced
- 2 tablespoons chili powder
- ½ teaspoon ground chipotle pepper
- ½ teaspoon ground cumin
- Salt to taste
- 3 ½ cups vegetable stock
- 1 15- ounce cans black beans rinsed
- 1 14.5- ounce can diced tomatoes
- ½ cup dried quinoa
- 4 teaspoons lime juice
- For serving: avocado cilantro, crema, cheese

Instructions

1. Heat a large heavy bottom pot with the oil over medium high heat.
2. Add the sweet potato and onion and cook for about 5 minutes, until the onion if softened.
3. Add the garlic, chili powder, chipotle, cumin and salt and stir to combine.
4. Add the stock, tomatoes, black beans and quinoa and bring the mixture to a boil. Stir everything to combine.
5. Cover the pot and reduce the heat to maintain a gentle simmer.
6. Cook for 30-40 minutes until the quinoa is fully cooked and the sweet potatoes are soft and the entire mixture is slightly thick like a chili.
7. Add the lime juice and remove the pot from the heat. Season with salt as needed.
8. Garnish with avocado, cilantro, crema or cheese before serving.

Nutrition Facts

Calories: 389kcal | Carbohydrates: 42g | Protein: 17g | Fat: 14g | Fiber: 9g | Sugar: 3g

Savory High-Protein Coconut Lentil Curry

Ready in 50 minutes

Servings: 6

Ingredients

- 2 tablespoons coconut oil
- 1 tablespoon each: cumin seeds and coriander seeds
- 1 head of garlic, chopped (10–12 cloves)
- 1 28-ounce can of crushed tomatoes
- 2 tablespoons ginger, chopped
- 1 tablespoon turmeric
- 2 teaspoons sea salt
- 1 cup dried brown lentils
- 1–2 teaspoons cayenne powder, optional
- 1 15-ounce can coconut milk
- A few handfuls of cherry tomatoes
- 1 cup chopped cilantro

Instructions

1. Heat the coconut oil in a large pot or skillet over medium-high heat. Add the cumin and coriander seeds and toast until they start to brown, about a minute. Add the garlic to the pot and let it brown, about 2 minutes.
2. Add the can of crushed tomatoes, ginger, turmeric, and sea salt to the pot and cook, stirring the pot a few times, for 5 minutes. Add the lentils and, if using, the cayenne powder, and 3 cups of water to the pot and bring it to a boil. Reduce the heat to low, cover the pot, and let it simmer for 35-40 minutes, or until the lentils are soft. Stir the pot a few times to prevent the lentils from sticking to the bottom. If the curry starts to look dry, add an extra 1/2 – 1 cup of water.
3. Once the lentils are soft, add the coconut milk and cherry tomatoes and bring the pot back to a simmer. Remove the pot from the heat and stir in the cilantro.

Nutrition Facts

Calories 266 | Total Fat 10g | Saturated Fat 4g | Cholesterol 0mg | Sodium 802mg | Total Carbohydrate 35g | Dietary Fiber 7g | Sugars 4g | Protein 11g

Skillet Potato and Tempeh Hash

Ready in 40 minutes

Servings: 4-6

Ingredients

- 4 medium to medium-large potatoes
- 2 tablespoons olive oil
- 1 medium onion, finely chopped
- 1 medium green or red bell pepper, finely diced
- 8-ounce package tempeh, any variety, finely diced
- 1 teaspoon all-purpose salt-free seasoning
- 1 teaspoon sweet or smoked paprika
- 1 cup kale, stemmed and finely chopped
- 1 to 2 tablespoons nutritional yeast, optional
- Salt and freshly ground pepper to taste
- Sriracha or other hot sauce for passing around

Instructions

1. Bake or microwave the potatoes ahead of time until done but still firm. If you'd like to leave the skins on, scrub them well. When cool enough to handle, finely dice them.
2. Heat the oil in a large skillet. Add the onion and sauté over medium heat until translucent. Add the bell pepper, tempeh, and potatoes. Turn the heat up to medium-high, and continue to sauté until all are turning golden brown. Stir frequently.
3. Add the seasonings and kale. Continue to cook, stirring frequently, until the mixture touched with brown spots here and there. If the skillet becomes dry, add a small amount of water, just enough to keep from sticking.
4. Stir in the nutritional yeast if using, and season with salt and pepper. Serve at once; pass around hot sauce for topping individual servings.

Nutrition Facts

Serving: 1 bowl | Calories: 269 | Total fat: 8g | Protein: 9g | Fiber: 6g | Carbs: 44g | Sodium: 18mg

The Vegan Buddha Bowl

Ready in 40 minutes

Servings: 2

Ingredients

Quinoa

- 1 Cup Quinoa rinsed
- 2 Cups Water

Chickpeas

- 1 1/2 Cups Cooked Chickpeas
- Drizzle Olive Oil or other neutral oil
- 1/2 Tsp Salt
- 1/2 Tsp Smoked Paprika
- 1 Tsp Chili Powder
- 1/8 Tsp Turmeric
- 1/2 Tsp Oregano

Red Pepper Sauce

- 1 Red Bell Pepper ribs and seeds removed
- 2 Tbs Olive Oil or other neutral oil
- Juice from 1/2 Lemon or more to taste
- 1/2 Tsp Pepper
- 1/2 Tsp Salt
- 1/2 Tsp Paprika
- 1/4 Cup Fresh Cilantro

For Serving

- Mixed Greens
- An Avocado
- Sesame Seeds for Garnish

Instructions

1. Firstly, cook the quinoa. Bring 2 cups water to a boil, then add quinoa. Simmer for about 15 minutes until all water is absorbed. When done, remove from heat and keep covered for about 10 minutes so quinoa can absorb any excess water.
2. Preheat oven to 425F. In a bowl, toss chickpeas, oil, and spices until chickpeas are evenly coated. On a baking sheet lined with parchment paper, bake chickpeas for 15-20 minutes, or until desired doneness is reached. When done, remove from oven and let cool.
3. To make red pepper dressing, add all dressing ingredients to a blender (not a food processor) and blend on high until smooth. Taste, and adjust seasonings to your preference.
4. Finally, assemble the buddha bowls. In two bowls, add quinoa, mixed greens, avocado, and chickpeas. Drizzle everything with red pepper sauce, and sprinkle with sesame seeds.

Nutrition Facts

Serving: 1 bowl | Calories 396 | Total Fat 16g | Saturated Fat 2g | Sodium 973mg | Total Carbohydrate 41g | Dietary Fiber 11g | Sugars 11g | Protein 21g

Sesame Soba Noodles with Collard Greens and Tempeh Croutons

Ready in 35 minutes

Servings: 4

Ingredients

Sauce

- ⅓ cup tahini
- ¼ cup lime juice
- 2 tablespoons reduced-sodium natural soy sauce or tamari, or more if needed
- 2 tablespoons natural granulated sugar (cane, coconut, or date) or agave nectar

Tempeh croutons

- 2 teaspoons dark sesame oil
- 1 tablespoon reduced-sodium natural soy sauce or tamari
- 1 package (8 ounces) tempeh, any variety, cut into ½" dice

Noodles

- 1 package (8 ounces) soba (buckwheat) noodles
- 10 to 12 collard green leaves
- 1 tablespoon dark sesame oil
- 1 large red or yellow onion, cut in half and thinly sliced
- ¼ small head green cabbage, cut into long, narrow shreds
- 1 medium red bell pepper, cut into long, narrow strips
- ½ cup chopped fresh cilantro, basil, or Thai basil leaves, or more as desired
- 1 tablespoon black or tan sesame seeds Red-pepper flakes or Sriracha sauce

Instructions

2. Make the sauce: In a small bowl, combine the tahini, lime juice, soy sauce or tamari, and sugar or agave nectar.
3. Make the croutons: In a large or wide-bottomed skillet, heat the oil and soy sauce or tamari over medium heat. Add the tempeh and stir to coat. Increase the heat to medium-high and cook the tempeh until most sides are golden brown. Remove the tempeh croutons to a plate.
4. Make the noodles: Cook the noodles according to package directions. When they're al dente, remove from the heat and drain.
5. Meanwhile, cut the stems from the collard leaves with kitchen shears or a sharp knife. Stack 6 or so halves of leaves at a time. Roll the leaves up tightly from one of the narrow ends, almost like a cigar shape, then thinly slice them. Let them unroll to create ribbons of collard greens. Give them a good rinse in a colander.
6. In the same skillet used to make the croutons, heat the oil. Add the onion and cook over medium heat until softened and golden. Add the collard ribbons, cover, and cook for 7 to 8 minutes, or until they wilt down a bit. Add the cabbage and bell pepper. Increase the heat and cook for 3 minutes, or just until the veggies are on the other side of raw. Remove the skillet from the heat.
7. Add the cooked noodles to the pan and use a large fork to mix the noodles thoroughly with the veggies. Pour the sauce over the mixture. Add the cilantro or basil and sesame seeds. Scatter the croutons on top. Season with the pepper flakes or Sriracha to taste. This can be served warm or at room temperature.

Nutrition Facts

Calories: 406kcal | Carbohydrates: 38g | Protein: 21g | Fat: 12g | Saturated Fat: 3g | Sodium: 621mg | Fiber: 7g | Sugar: 6g

Vegan Chow Mein with Zucchini Noodles and Tofu

Ready in 30 minutes

Servings: 4

Ingredients

Marinade

- 13 oz extra firm tofu drained, cut into cubes
- 2 Tbsp gluten free tamari
- 1 Tbsp rice wine vinegar
- 1 Tbsp fresh grated ginger
- 1/2 tsp sesame oil
- 1/2 tsp Vegetable Better Than Bouillon
- 1 1/2 Tbsp coconut sugar

Sauce

- 1 tsp Vegetable Better Than Bouillon
- 2 Tbsp tamari gluten free tamari
- 1 Tbsp rice wine vinegar
- 1 Tbsp fresh grated ginger
- 1/2 tsp sesame oil
- 1 1/2 tbsp coconut sugar
- 1 Tbsp gluten free hoisin sauce
- 1 Tbsp cornstarch

Stir-Fry

- 2 tsp coconut oil divided
- 2 carrots spiralized
- 1 cup broccoli cut into small florets
- 4 zucchini spiralized
- 2 baby bok choy sliced lengthwise
- 1 bell pepper julienne
- 8 oz cremini mushrooms thinly sliced

- A pinch salt and pepper pinch of each
- 1 cup bean sprouts
- 1 scallion sliced thinly on a bias
- White and black sesame seeds for garnish

Instructions

1. Line a plate with paper towels, add the tofu pieces and top with another few layers of paper towels. Add a plate and something heavy (like a few cookbooks) and press the moisture out of the tofu.
2. Meanwhile, in a large bowl, mix together the marinade ingredients and transfer to a sealable plastic bag. Add in the pressed tofu and allow the tofu to marinate in the fridge for 1-2 hours.
3. When ready to cook, mix together the sauce ingredients in a bowl and set aside.
4. Add 1 teaspoon of the coconut oil to a nonstick skillet and cook the tofu over medium high heat until golden brown on all sides, about 4-5 minutes. Remove from the pan and set aside.
5. Wipe out the pan (to prevent the marinade from burning), add in the remaining teaspoon of oil and heat to medium high. Add the carrots and broccoli and allow to cook for 2-3 minutes. Then add in the zucchini, bok choy, bell pepper, cremini mushrooms and a pinch each of salt and pepper. The salt will help to draw out the moisture so it can start to evaporate. Allow the veggies to cook for 5 minutes, making sure to toss everything frequently.
6. Add in the sauce, and again, toss to coat. Cook until the sauce thickens, and the vegetables reach a nice al dente stage.
7. Finally, add in the bean sprouts and the tofu to rewarm and mix everything together once more. Season with salt and pepper, if desired, to taste.
8. When ready to serve, pile the tofu on top of the vegetables and noodles, top with the scallion and sesame seeds and enjoy!

Nutrition Facts

Calories: 310kcal | Carbohydrates: 35g | Protein: 10g | Fat: 4g

High-Protein Cauliflower Rice Burrito Bowl

Ready in 30 minutes

Servings: 3 bowls

Ingredients

Beans

- 1 15-ounce can black or pinto beans
- 1/2 tsp ground cumin
- 1/2 tsp chili powder
- Salt to taste

Cauliflower Rice

- 1 Tbsp olive or grape seed oil
- 3 cloves garlic, minced
- 1/4 cup diced red or white onion
- 1 medium head cauliflower, grated
- 1 pinch sea salt
- 3 Tbsp lime juice
- 1 tsp ground cumin
- 1/2 tsp chili powder
- 1/3 cup red or green salsa
- 1/4 cup fresh chopped cilantro

Peppers + Onions

- 1 Tbsp olive or grape seed oil
- 1 medium red, green, orange, or yellow bell pepper (thinly sliced lengthwise)
- 1/2 medium red onion, sliced into rings
- 1 pinch sea salt

Instructions

1. Add beans to a small saucepan over medium heat and season with spices to taste. Bring to a boil, then reduce heat to low and stir occasionally.
2. Grate cauliflower. Then heat a large rimmed skillet over medium heat.
3. Once hot, add oil, garlic, onion, and a pinch each salt and pepper. Sauté for 1 minute, stirring frequently. Then add cauliflower 'rice' and stir to coat.
4. Place the lid on to steam the rice for about 2-4 minutes or until almost tender like rice (al dente in texture), stirring occasionally. Chop up your bell pepper and onion at this time.
5. Remove rice from heat and transfer to a large mixing bowl. Add lime juice, cumin, chili powder, salsa and fresh cilantro. Stir to combine and set aside.
6. Heat the large skillet back over medium-high heat. Once hot, add oil, bell pepper and onion and a pinch of sea salt. Sauté, stirring frequently, until slightly softened and they take on a little color - about 4 minutes.
7. To serve, divide rice, beans, and peppers between serving bowls. Enjoy as is or with corn tortillas, chips, salsa, lime juice, hot sauce, or guacamole.

Nutrition Facts

Serving: 1 bowl | Calories: 269kcal | Carbohydrates: 44g | Protein: 15g | Fat: 15g | Saturated Fat: 2.2g | Sodium: 195mg | Fiber: 12g | Sugar: 3,5g

Vegetarian Slow Cooker Lentil Sloppy Joes with Spaghetti Squash

Ready in 4 hours

Servings: 4

Ingredients

- 1 1/4 cups uncooked green lentils, rinsed and drained
- 1 white onion, finely diced
- 1 red pepper, finely diced
- 1 carrot, thinly sliced (carrot is optional)
- 3 cloves garlic, minced
- 1 1/2 tablespoons chili powder
- 1 teaspoon cumin
- 1/2 teaspoon onion powder
- 1/4 teaspoon cayenne pepper
- 1 - (15 oz) can tomato sauce
- 1 - (15 oz) can diced tomatoes
- 1 1/2 cups water, plus more if necessary
- 2 tablespoons organic ketchup
- 1 teaspoon yellow mustard
- 1 teaspoon gluten free soy sauce
- 1 spaghetti squash, washed
- Salt and pepper, to taste

Instructions

1. In a large slow cooker, add in all ingredients except spaghetti squash. Stir to combine.
2. Cut the washed spaghetti squash in half around the middle and scoop out the seeds. Place the squash halves face down in the slow cooker right on top of the lentils. Cover and cook on high for 4 hours or until squash is tender and lentils are cooked completely. If the lentils seem dry in any way, just stir in some water until it reaches a nice thick, consistency.

3. Remove spaghetti squash and shred inside with a fork. Divide among bowls and add lentil sloppy joe topping. Sprinkle with cheese, if desired.

Nutrition Facts

Serving: 1 bowl | Calories: 358kcal | Fat: 3g | Carbohydrates: 67g | Fiber: 14g | Sugar: 12g | Protein: 16g

Chickpea, Tofu, and Eggplant Curry

Ready in 40 minutes

Servings: 4

Ingredients

- 2 tablespoons coconut oil, divided
- 1 package of medium-firm tofu, cubed and dried with paper towel
- 1 long Asian eggplants, quartered into 3-inch strips
- 1/2 large onion, very thinly sliced
- 1 tablespoons minced ginger
- 1 garlic cloves, minced
- 1 tablespoon garam masala
- 1/2 tablespoon each: cumin seeds, turmeric, sea salt
- 1/4 cup tomato paste
- 1 can coconut milk
- 1/2 can water
- 1 15-ounce can chickpeas, drained and rinsed
- Cilantro, to serve

Instructions

1. Heat 1/2 tablespoon of the coconut oil in a large, non-stick frying pan over medium-high heat. Add the tofu and pan fry until golden brown on 2 sides, about 5 minutes. Remove from the pan and set aside.
2. Heat 1 tablespoon of coconut oil in the pan used for the tofu. Brown the eggplant on all sides, working in batches if needed. Remove the eggplant from the pan.
3. Heat the remaining 1/2 tablespoon of coconut oil in the same pan used for the eggplant. Add the onion and cook for 2-3 minutes, or until it softens. Add the ginger and garlic and cook for 1 minute. Add the garam masala, cumin seeds, and turmeric to the pan and let them toast for 1 minute, stirring constantly. Add the sea salt and the tomato paste and cook for 1 minute, stirring constantly.
4. Add the coconut milk and water to the pot, bring it to a boil and stir, scraping the bottom for any stuck on bits. Add the eggplant back into

the pan and turn the heat to low. Let the eggplant cook, uncovered, for 12-15 minutes, or until it is soft but not mushy.
5. Stir the chickpeas and tofu into the curry and let them heat through. Serve with some rice (or, my favorite, cauliflower rice) and some cilantro on top.

Nutrition Facts

Calories: 536kcal | Carbohydrates: 49g | Protein: 21g | Fat: 35g | Saturated Fat: 7g | Sodium: 549mg | Potassium: 928mg | Fiber: 18g | Sugar: 6g

Roasted Teriyaki Mushrooms and Broccolini Soba Noodles

Ready in 30 minutes

Servings: 4

Ingredients

Mushrooms

- 3 8 oz containers of button mushrooms
- 1 tbsp high heat oil
- 1 tbsp rice wine vinegar
- 1 tbsp honey
- 1 tbsp tamari (gluten free soy sauce) or soy sauce
- 1 tsp grated ginger
- Soba Noodles with Vegetables
- 1 package of gluten free buckwheat soba noodles
- 1 tbs olive oil
- 2 cloves garlic, minced
- ½ shallot, diced
- 2 bunches broccolini, ends cut off and if the stems are thick cut them in half lengthwise
- 1 stalk kale, cut into shreds

Sauce

- ¼ cup tamari (gluten free soy sauce) or soy sauce
- 2 tablespoons olive oil
- Juice of 1 lemon
- 1 tablespoon toasted sesame oil
- 1 tablespoon honey
- 1 teaspoon sriracha
- 1 tsp grated ginger

Instructions

1. Preheat oven to 425 and line a baking sheet with parchment paper.

2. Trim stems off the mushrooms, cut each mushroom in half, and place them in a large bowl.
3. In another bowl whisk together the mushroom glaze ingredients. Pour the glaze over the mushrooms in a bowl and mix until all the mushrooms are evenly coated. Pour the mushrooms onto the parchment lined baking sheet and place them in the preheated oven for 15 minutes. Remove and toss so they cook evenly. Roast for another 15 minutes.
4. Meanwhile, cook soba noodles according to package directions and heat a large skillet with 1 tbs olive oil over medium heat. Add minced garlic and diced shallot and cook for 1 minute. Add broccolini, kale, and salt and pepper to taste, and cook until just tender, about 5 minutes.
5. While vegetables and noodles are cooking, whisk together the soba noodle sauce ingredients in a bowl.
6. Add cooked noodles to the pan of broccolini and kale, add the sauce, and stir until all the vegetables and noodles are evenly coated in sauce.
7. Place a portion of noodles and vegetables into bowls and top them with the roasted mushroom. Garnish with sesame seeds, hot peppers, and green onions.

Nutrition Facts

Calories: 406kcal | Carbohydrates: 35g | Protein: 16g | Fat: 12g | Saturated Fat: 3g | Sodium: 621mg | Fiber: 7g | Sugar: 6g

High-Protein Soup & Stew Recipes

Lentil Spinach Soup

Ready in 45 minutes

Servings: 4 bowls

Ingredients

- 1 medium onion, chopped
- 1-2 small carrots
- 1 clove garlic, minced
- 1 cup green/brown lentils (uncooked)
- 15 oz. can diced tomatoes
- 1 cups vegetable broth
- 1 oz. spinach
- 1 tsp. cumin
- 1/2 tsp. smoked paprika
- Salt to taste

Instructions

1. Dice onion and carrot.
2. In a stockpot over medium-high heat, saute onion and carrot for about 7 minutes.
3. Meanwhile, mince garlic and rinse lentils.
4. Add garlic, cumin, smoked paprika, and salt to stockpot. Saute 1 minute.
5. Add broth, tomatoes, and lentils. Increase heat and bring to a boil.
6. Reduce heat, cover, and simmer for about 30 minutes or until lentils are tender.
7. Meanwhile, roughly chop spinach.
8. Add spinach during last couple minutes of cooking.
9. Salt to taste.

Nutrition Facts

Calories: 231kcal | Carbohydrates: 42g | Protein: 17g | Fat: 1g | Potassium: 910mg | Fiber: 17g | Sugar: 7g | Vitamin A: 5505IU | Vitamin C: 21.6mg | Calcium: 108mg | Iron: 6.3mg

Extremely Delicious Lentil Soup

Ready in 50 minutes

Servings: 4

Ingredients

- ¼ cup extra virgin olive oil
- 1 medium yellow or white onion, chopped
- 1 large carrot, peeled and chopped
- 1 garlic clove, pressed or minced
- 2 teaspoons ground cumin
- 1 teaspoon curry powder
- ½ teaspoon dried thyme
- 1 large can (28 ounces) diced tomatoes, lightly drained
- 1 cup brown or green lentils, picked over and rinsed
- 1 cup vegetable broth
- 2 cups water
- 1 teaspoon salt, more to taste
- Pinch of red pepper flakes
- Freshly ground black pepper, to taste
- 1 cup chopped fresh collard greens or kale, tough ribs removed
- 1 to 2 tablespoons lemon juice (½ to 1 medium lemon), to taste

Instructions

1. Heat the olive oil in a large Dutch oven or pot over medium heat. One-fourth cup olive oil may seem like a lot, but it adds a lovely richness and heartiness to this nutritious soup.
2. Once the oil is shimmering, add the chopped onion and carrot and cook, stirring often, until the onion has softened and is turning translucent, about 5 minutes.
3. Add the garlic, cumin, curry powder and thyme. Cook until fragrant while stirring constantly, about 30 seconds. Pour in the drained diced tomatoes and cook for a few more minutes, stirring often, in order to enhance their flavor.

4. Pour in the lentils, broth and the water. Add 1 teaspoon salt and a pinch of red pepper flakes. Season generously with freshly ground black pepper. Raise heat and bring the mixture to a boil, then partially cover the pot and reduce the heat to maintain a gentle simmer. Cook for 25 to 30 minutes, or until the lentils are tender but still hold their shape.
5. Transfer 2 cups of the soup to a blender. Securely fasten the lid, protect your hand from steam with a tea towel placed over the lid, and purée the soup until smooth. Pour the puréed soup back into the pot.
6. Add the chopped greens and cook for 5 more minutes, or until the greens have softened to your liking. Remove the pot from the heat and stir in 1 tablespoon of lemon juice. Taste and season with more salt, pepper and/or lemon juice until the flavors really sing. For spicier soup, add another pinch or two of red pepper flakes.

Nutrition Facts

Serving: 1 bowl | Calories 366 | Total Fat 16g | Saturated Fat 2g | Trans Fat 0g | Polyunsaturated Fat 2g | Monounsaturated Fat 10g | Cholesterol 0mg | Sodium 1376mg | Total Carbohydrate 48g | Dietary Fiber 11g | Sugars 11g | Protein 17g

Sweet Potato, Spinach & Butter Bean Stew

Ready in 45 minutes

Servings: 3

Ingredients

- 1 pound sweet potatoes
- 9 oz young leaf spinach
- 4 x 14 oz can chopped tomatoes
- 2 x 14 oz can butter beans
- 4 garlic cloves, crushed
- 2 medium onions (finely chopped)
- 2 Tbsp olive oil
- 2 tsp ground cumin
- 2 tsp ground coriander
- 3 tsp smoked paprika
- 3 cups vegetable stock
- Juice of 1 to 2 lemons
- Large bunch of fresh coriander
- Salt & pepper to taste

Instructions

1. Peel sweet potatoes and cut in 1/2-inch.
1. Heat olive oil in a large casserole pan. Add finely chopped onion, crushed garlic, ground cumin, ground coriander and smoked paprika. Cook until onion is soft.
2. Add diced sweet potatoes, chopped tomatoes and stock.
3. Bring to the boil, then cook half covered until sweet potatoes are tender
4. Stir in spinach. Cook for 2 minutes. Add rinsed and drained butter beans. Cook for another 2 minutes to warm them through.
5. Season to taste with lemon juice, salt & pepper.
6. Serve with plenty of chopped fresh coriander leaves sprinkled over.

Nutrition Facts

Calories: 430kcal | Carbohydrates: 41g | Protein: 15g | Fat: 8g | Saturated Fat: 3g | Cholesterol: 11mg | Sodium: 533mg

Pressure Cooker Pea Soup

Ready in 40 minutes

Servings: 6-8

Ingredients

- 1 pound dried split peas
- 1 medium-sized onion, diced
- 2 stalks celery, diced
- 8 cups water
- 1 teaspoon dried thyme
- 3 garlic cloves, minced
- A pinch ground black pepper
- 1 teaspoon salt
- 1 teaspoon hot pepper sauce (I prefer Tabasco)

Instructions

1. Pour water into your pressure cooker. Add split peas, diced onion, celery, thyme, minced garlic, and black pepper.
2. Close the pressure cooker lid securely and place pressure regulator over vent according to manufacturer's instructions. Bring to a high pressure and cook about 30 minutes.
3. When the timer beeps, reduce the pressure using a natural method.
4. Open the lid and stir well to distribute flavors.
5. Season with salt and hot pepper sauce and serve hot. You may also top the soup with chopped parsley or cilantro.

Nutrition Facts

Calories: 430kcal | Carbohydrates: 41g | Protein: 15g | Fat: 8g | Saturated Fat: 3g | Cholesterol: 11mg | Sodium: 533mg

Conclusion

Thank you for downloading my book and taking the time to learn new Vegan recipes.

I hope that my High-Protein Cookbook for Athletes allows you to cook delicious and healthy plant-based meals and create the body of your dream.

Thank you again and be healthy!

Made in the USA
Columbia, SC
04 February 2025